C000065216

THE
NATURAL
—— WAY TO ——
STOP
SNORING

THE
NATURAL
— WAY TO —
STOP
SNORING

Dr Elizabeth Scott

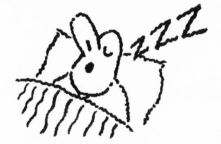

ORION

An Orion paperback
First published in Great Britain in 1995 by Orion
an imprint of Orion Books Ltd,
Orion House, 5 Upper St Martin's Lane, London WC2H 9EA

A CIP catalogue record for this book is available from the
British Library.

ISBN: 0 75280 067 1

Typeset by Deltatype Ltd, Ellesmere Port, Cheshire
Printed and bound in Great Britain by
Clays Ltd, St Ives plc

Contents

Introduction

Who says you snore? Your bed partner? You had better believe it. Let her use a tape recorder if you doubt it and a recording of you snoring, with its snorts and starts, will soon convince you that whatever you thought you were doing all night, you were not enjoying sound, refreshing sleep.

Why shouldn't you snore if you want to?

Because snoring, whatever its cause, is not a normal or healthy way to breathe and by itself will deprive you and your partner of a good night's sleep. In addition, it may be the first sign that you are on the way to getting a more severe problem, the obstructive sleep apnoea/ hypopnoea syndrome (SAHS), where your upper throat blocks as you snore and you wake, or almost wake, with a snort. This may happen to you up to 300 times a night. These repeated breath stoppages begin to cause a lack of oxygen in the brain and other vital organs of your body. Your sleep pattern is disrupted and your health seriously threatened by SAHS.

But snoring, by itself, causes the malaise that accompanies chronic sleep deprivation in you and in your partner. If you are a serious snorer, or have your sleep disrupted by a snorer, you are likely to wake with a headache and feel tired, especially in the mornings. You will get easily despondent and depressed about minor problems and lack the energy you used to have to tackle your day's work. Your daytime concentration is so poor that when you are driving you are at increased risk of having an accident.

Is this you?

If so, this book is for you.

If you have gained weight and are heavier than you ought to be; if your collar size is over seventeen and your nights are restless due to your repeated awakenings, you may well be in the early stages of obstructive sleep apnoea. It predisposes its sufferers to heart disease and strokes and in Great Britain it affects up to four per cent of middle-aged men and two per cent of middle-aged women.

In the USA, perhaps because there are more sleep assessment centres, the number of diagnosed SAHS patients is even higher. Now that doctors realize that obstructive sleep apnoea has these serious consequences, they are more likely to look for it among their patients.

Snoring is something you should not ignore. Doctors have paid little attention to it because they have not had a quick cure handy. But obstructive sleep apnoea has been recognized as an illness since 1877, when Dr Broadbent of St Mary's Hospital in London described a patient of his who snored heavily and who had recurrent obstruction of his breathing on inspiration while asleep. (Mr Pickwick, a fat, sleepy person who snored heavily and whose daytime was made miserable by poor concentration, headaches and increasing gloom, was a typical sufferer from sleep apnoea.)

What doctors are finding now is that there are many more people who have sleep apnoea in a less acute form, sufficient to make their working day a misery and to put them at risk of the increase in cardiac and respiratory problems that accompany long-term sleep apnoea.

Doctors are no longer shy of diagnosing the problem. Their difficulty comes when they have to treat this common affliction.

Introduction

The only non-surgical relief they will offer you at present is to sleep with a face mask attached to a constant positive airways pressure machine, which keeps your upper airway open. No one wants to sleep with a machine. Yet once your snoring has been established as being serious enough to warrant the diagnosis of sleep apnoea, you will be given no choice.

These 'CPAP' machines sit, purring away on the bedside table, attached to a tube and face mask for you to wear while asleep. They deliver air at a slightly raised pressure, which holds the upper throat and airway open. This may be acceptable for those grossly obese elderly people whose very lives are threatened by the poor circulating blood-oxygen levels that accompany sleep apnoea, but I see this prescription as a life sentence. Using a condom is one thing, but taking off a face mask, switching off a machine and cleaning up your sweaty face before sex is more like disassembling the mechanical man. It is a turn off.

But you don't want to feel tired all day either, or to have the guilt of keeping your partner awake. So, for those of you who, like me, want to feel a little bit younger, a little bit fitter, I have devised a set of exercises to widen and strengthen your upper throat and tone up your soft palate. If the problem is a deterioration in the musculature and size of your upper throat area, holding it open with a machine is a confession of failure. It seems more sensible to allow you to work your muscles in this area till they are as strong as they used to be before you started snoring, and to widen your upper throat area as it was before you gained weight.

Specialists may feel that once the brain has been starved of oxygen for long enough it is impossible to recover from sleep apnoea. I can only say that I have seen patients with proven sleep apnoeic episodes and loud snoring lose both these symptoms with weight loss and exercises for their upper throat.

I have been Senior Partner in a General Practice in Edinburgh for over twenty-five years and in this time I have seen the ill health that sleep loss of all kinds engenders. Snorers and their partners suffer, but up till recently I had no reasonable treatment to offer them.

When I became the Honorary Medical Adviser to the Scottish Chamber Orchestra, I came in contact not only with instrumentalists, but singers. It was seeing professional singers and realizing that they seldom snored that spurred me to see if they were doing something that other people do not. Of course they were.

They all performed regular exercises to widen their upper throats and increase the power of their soft palates. Just the thing to prevent snoring.

My exercises are based on their regular, upper throat 'work-out'. Like all self-help treatments, it is hard work; but the reward is great.

Chapter One

What Happens When You Go to Sleep

Anatomists have known for years about how the tissues of your throat are formed and function, but it is really only in the last sixty years that they have been able to find out what happens to you, and particularly what happens in your brain, when you sleep. The great breakthrough was the invention of the electro-encephalograph, which records electrical impulses given off by the brain through electrodes placed on your head. This non-invasive, painless process showed the world that sleep, far from being a mini death, was a time of furious activity within your brain as well as a time of tissue renewal in your body. The old wives' recommendation, 'A good sleep and you'll feel better' is, as usual, being endorsed by scientists years after everyone knew about it from experience.

You have all watched a baby sleep. Very young ones drift in and out of rapid eye movement sleep, where their bodies lie relaxed and their eyes move behind their lids. During their first three months, babies spend more time in rapid eye movement sleep than in deep, non-rapid eye movement sleep. This makes sense when you realize that during these months baby remains very helpless physically but his or her brain and nervous system are developing at a great rate to reach a more adult state. The brain centres controlling rapid eye movement sleep therefore switch off the normal messages that activate the limbs and major muscles of posture so that the blood circulation to the brain can be increased in order that the cells in the brain can have the oxygen supply they need to mature. Baby lies immobile while his or her brain gets on with growing up.

This is the part of sleep where you will snore worst, for the same reason: your body muscles are completely relaxed and the lax tissues in the upper throat area vibrate in the inspired air and may block your upper throat.

To understand exactly what happens, I want to describe the stages of normal sleep as you can see it charted by an electro-encephalograph.

When you close your eyes and drift into sleep, the low irregular alpha waves, which occur when you are awake, slow to low-voltage, flattish waves which run at about 6 cycles per second. You are then said to be in stage 1 non-rapid eye movement sleep. You all know this stage; it occurs when you nod off in a boring lecture. Odd thoughts and fancies invade your mind and you drift away so gently from reality that waking produces a feeling of surprise. (I remember one long, tiring dinner party where, ensconced on a lush sofa, I surfaced with the firm statement, 'I believe the fat content of Red Poll milk is 4 per cent.' My hostess, who was offering me cream for my coffee, was clearly not prepared for that answer, and in fact looked as if she had just asked me something quite different.) Stage 1 non-REM sleep can give you a reputation for eccentricity.

If you are undisturbed, your sleep deepens.

In stage 2 non-rapid eye movement sleep, the brain wave rate slows further and on the electro-encephalograph small 'spindles' of rapidly increasing and decreasing waves occur suddenly. 'K complexes', where a sudden, single, high wave complex is seen, are also typical of this stage of sleep. These interruptions of the normal wave pattern are often due to noises or internal disturbance, where waking almost occurs.

If you continue undisturbed, your sleep deepens still further and large slow waves of 2 cycles per second or less develop. When these occupy over 20 per cent of the electro-encephalograph tracing, stage 3 non-REM sleep is said to be present, and when they occur over 50 per cent of the time, stage 4 non-REM sleep has supervened.

It is in these deep stages of non-rapid eye movement sleep that growth hormone is released. This stimulates growth in children and tissue regeneration in adults whose growth has stopped. This deep sleep is an essential part of keeping your body healthy.

Those of you who snore are wakened by the noise, or are almost aroused, again and again through the night. You are allowed no reasonable time in deep, restorative sleep.

If you have that more serious form of snoring, sleep apnoea, when your throat is repeatedly blocked by your soft palate falling back and you suffer the choking that is so typical of this condition, it ensures you are not only deprived of enough deep non-REM sleep to rejuvenate the body, but in REM sleep the loss of oxygen to the brain can be positively damaging.

Your sleep–wake cycle is controlled by centres deep in the brain stem, the hypothalamus and basal forebrain, those more primitive parts of the brain that are intrinsic to life. A circadian rhythm controls your waking and sleeping through the twenty-four hours you call 'one day'. It organizes your temperature to remain steady through the morning, drop slightly in the early afternoon, when you feel sleepy, and then rise again for the rest of the day. When you go to bed at night your temperature again falls to reach an all-time low when you are most deeply asleep, thereafter rising slowly throughout the rest of the night to your wakening in the morning. In the late stages of the night, cortisol and prolactin are secreted. These hormones act as a sort of morning boost to wakening, a natural equivalent to the drive you get from that first morning cup of tea or coffee.

Throughout your twenty-four hours you also experience the effects of your ultradian rhythm clock, so called because, in contrast to the circadian rhythm, it occurs more than once a day. It is your ultradian rhythm that tends to make you hungry or restless every 90 to 120 minutes. The presence of this rhythmic control is easily confirmed during the day by your feelings of being able to concentrate on one subject for only this length of time before you need a break or something to eat. It also occurs through the night, as the electro-encephalograph shows. You move from sleep stage to sleep stage every 1½ to 2 hours through the night, first diving into the deep stages of non-REM sleep, which you may reach within twenty minutes of falling asleep.

After sliding into deep non-REM sleep for about an hour and a half, your sleep lightens and you may return to stage 2 sleep, with its spindles and K complexes. From here your sleep may deepen if your body needs it, or you may move into rapid eye movement sleep, when you usually experience dreams.

REM sleep seems to be for the brain. It is controlled by centres in the brain stem which in turn control the circulation of blood to the brain, which is greatly increased. At the same time, these centres switch off the nerve signals from the motor areas of the cortex to the body muscles so that they lie atonic and paralysed. The only muscles that remain mobile are those of the eyes and eyebrow area and the diaphragm, that great muscle that separates the chest from the abdomen and is one of the main muscles of breathing.

The diaphragm acts as a piston so that your body continues to get oxygen into the lungs, although breathing in this stage may become quite irregular.

It is mainly in this REM stage that snoring is at its worst. The muscles of the upper throat and soft palate lie lax and atonic. The muscles between your ribs and around your shoulder girdle, which you usually use to help your diaphragm pull air into your lungs, lie paralysed. Although the brain may be getting a spring clean for the next day, the body is in a dangerously helpless state in REM sleep. (It has been suggested that some cot deaths may occur while baby is in rapid eye movement sleep, because if a blockage in his airway occurs he may not be as able to deal with it as he would when all his muscles are active.)

Snoring disrupts your airway and in sleep apnoea may totally obstruct it. Emergency signals wake you to muscular activity in order to breathe properly if your airway completely blocks. Your partner will hear you rouse with a snort as you suddenly pull air into your lungs.

Research suggests that when two people

sleep together they tend to go through the same stages of sleep at much the same time. This means that if you are not getting enough rapid eye movement sleep because of your snoring, not only is your brain getting short-changed by not getting the number of hours it needs in this stage of sleep which is specially for the brain, but your partner may also be suffering in the same way.

A snorer may be aroused, choking, out of REM sleep either into light sleep or wakening up to 300 times a night. This is not getting a good night's sleep.

Chapter Two

What Happens When
You Snore

When you snore, the sound is most often caused by the air you breathe in, vibrating your soft palate.

Look in a mirror and say 'Ah'. You can see the soft palate as a floppy extension of the hard palate which lies behind your upper teeth. It is formed by muscles like butterfly's wings that meet in the centre where they are attached to a tough, midline fibrous strap. When the muscles contract they pull the soft palate up and back to help to close off the upper throat and nose as food is swallowed.

In this endeavour the soft palate is assisted by the upper throat muscles, which lie round the upper throat like a hand gripping a tube. When they contract, they pull the throat forward and make it narrower. The uvula, that little muscular area hanging down from the middle of the soft palate, fills in any gaps.

Year after year, meal after meal this is what you use your soft palate, uvula and upper throat muscles for. You are about to swallow: tighten the upper throat; stop the food going up your nose.

This may have been enough to keep the muscles in strong working order when early man tore and tried to swallow tough pieces of meat and vegetable matter brought in from the hunt. It is not like that any more. Small wonder that, as you get older, put on weight and eat and drink the soft, processed food of developed countries, your upper throat muscles atrophy and fat gets laid down where muscle should be.

You can see this happen over your stomach from the age of about thirty-five onwards if you do not keep up a habit of vigorous exercise. If you are gaining fat over your stomach, it is being laid down everywhere and around your throat is no exception. Even if you practise food restriction, you may not put on weight but your stomach muscles get thinner and less strong. In the same way, the muscles around your throat and in your soft palate get thinner and frail, only just able to cope with their day-to-day function.

The fitness of muscle strength you have built in childhood and young adulthood no longer carries you along. You potter to work, potter after children; muscles atrophy. You seldom even sing and shout as you used to in school. Why expect your soft palate muscles and upper throat muscles to be other than vestigial valves, able only to help your food down and lie flaccid and toneless when you are asleep?

The soft palate is thus easy to vibrate as it is really mostly a fibrous central strap with a covering of fat; and the upper throat tends to lie semicontracted, ready to swallow but also constricting the passage of inspired air.

Does this matter? Not during the daytime, when the normal activity of your musculature can override any problems. However, when you are deep asleep in stage 3 or 4 non-rapid eye movement sleep, your relaxation may let your upper throat collapse inwards but, more important, when you are in rapid eye movement sleep all your muscles of posture, as well as your upper throat and soft palate muscles, lie almost paralysed. This is a fact that most people do not know and should. When you are in 'dream' sleep and the brain is attending to its own make and mend, it switches off signals to the limb muscles as well as to the ancillary muscles of breathing such as those between your ribs. All the upper throat and soft palate muscles lie in relaxed paralysis as well. Muscle in itself is a tough structure; even when flaccid it has its own strength. Fat has not. It flops where its weight takes it. If your soft palate and upper throat have become surrounded by fat, they are very vulnerable to collapse if there is any pressure change brought to bear. When this happens, your lack of intrinsic muscle tone matters a great deal.

Your snoring may not be so severe that your brain becomes short of oxygen, as happens in sleep apnoea, but every time you are half-woken by your snore, your blood pressure shoots up and settles, just as it does if you get a sudden surprise in the daytime. If your blood pressure is absolutely normal all that happens is that your heart does not get the rest it expects at night. This, over the years, is not going to do it any good. But say your blood pressure is borderline high because, perhaps, you have put on a bit of unnecessary weight. Your doctor is going to think that you will be lying peaceful all night, allowing your blood pressure to settle to its lowest level for at least eight hours in the twenty-four. He could not be more wrong. You will be getting spikes of higher pressure with each arousal right through the night.

When I am deciding whether to start a patient on medication to lower a blood pressure that is on the borderline of being too high, I always ask if he snores. It helps me to make up my mind whether he really needs the medication for life that treating high blood pressure entails.

So simple snoring can have a deleterious effect on your body. The trouble is that simple snoring tends to get worse. It is the first sign that your upper throat and soft palate have lost their intrinsic muscle strength. If your upper throat muscles have deteriorated this far, they are not going to get any better without regular and serious exercise. If the area around your upper throat and soft palate muscles is infiltrated by fat, then this also must go, just as to get fit, if you are overweight, you must lose your beer belly and change the fat laid down over your stomach to good contractile muscle. Without exercise, the upper throat and soft palate continue to weaken. You start to suffer from sleep apnoea, where the soft palate totally obstructs the upper throat. In sleep apnoea when you breathe in, during the deeper stages of non-REM sleep or more especially in

REM sleep when most of the muscles of respiration and throat lie flaccid, the air passes up the nose and, as it does so, the increase in resistance of the tissues it passes over leads to a loss of pressure in the upper part of the throat. Your lax soft palate is drawn into the stream of air and vibrated to produce snoring. Worse, your lax upper throat muscles, covered in fat, are pulled in to cause this part of the throat to narrow.

Your vibrating floppy soft palate now falls back to block the upper throat. No air gets through to the lungs. Your diaphragmatic muscle, the only one helping you breathe in REM sleep, strains against the blockage. You grunt as your diaphragm tries to pull air through the lungs. Nothing happens. You seem not to be breathing, as no air passes. You strain and grunt again and again until either the blockage is overcome by the diaphragm's muscular effort, or the concentration of carbon dioxide gathering in the brain so increases that you are woken. You either awake suddenly with a great snort as the air breaks through this barrier and the lungs are again filled with air, or you almost awake with a sharp rise in blood pressure and a gasp of oxygen-rich air pulled into your lungs.

This may happen again and again all night. At best you remain in the earlier stages of sleep. Any return to deeper stages or rapid eye movement sleep produces the same blockage. After some years of this, your brain may react so lethargically to oxygen deprivation that you scarcely struggle against it. Only in REM sleep, when there is sudden complete blockage, does acute wakening occur. The brain seems to react very promptly to oxygen lack in this stage of sleep, which appears to be particularly for brain care.

Sleep apnoea is made worse if you take sleeping pills which further dull the brain's response to poor oxygen supply. Over-indulgence in alcohol can have the same effect. Worse, if you continue to have this recurring blockage of air into the lungs, your brain becomes chronically oxygen-starved. Those with lung problems, such as asthma and chronic obstructive airways disease, are even more at risk from the problems associated with sleep apnoea. Being overweight helps neither the snorer nor those with sleep apnoea.

Not all snoring is due to a narrow throat and floppy soft palate. In relaxed sleep, when we breathe in, any lax tissue in the nose or upper throat that the air is pulled over will tend to vibrate, just as air blown over a clarinet reed or in a bagpipe chanter vibrates to give sound.

Some people snore because their nasal passages are blocked. Perhaps they have a deviated nasal septum or nasal polyps, which vibrate in the stream of inspired air. They may have a stuffy nose due to infection or an allergy such as hay fever. They may have enlarged adenoids lying behind the nasal passage, or large tonsils. They may have a goitre causing throat constriction further down, or a narrow larynx. Most of these rarer conditions are curable, medically or surgically.

Children who snore often have enlarged tonsils and adenoids, especially between the ages of three and seven, when these glands are at their largest. Snoring and their habit of sleeping in a knee/shoulder position (with their head bent back on their pillow and their knees drawn up under their abdomen) often makes their mother bring them to surgery to see what is wrong. They are simply trying to keep their upper airway open by bending their heads back.

However, most snorers snore because their upper throat is narrow and their soft palate musculature lax. These are the serious snorers because this condition, as it gets worse, leads to sleep apnoea. This sort of snoring is curable, I believe, with the exercises singers use to widen the upper throat and strengthen the soft palate.

This is just common sense. Where your throat is narrowed by fat deposits overlying contracted vestigial inactive muscle it is bound not to have the strength to withstand the pressure drop that occurs in the upper throat, especially during REM sleep. This picture will illustrate what is happening.

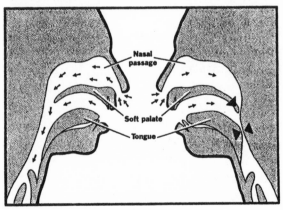

Collapse of upper airway due to increased nasal passage resistance and a floppy soft palate and upper throat.

But you can exercise this area so that you build the muscles surrounding your upper throat and make them elastic. You can widen this area with exercise helped by weight loss and the preferential loss of fat deposits that you get when you exercise a particular muscle area, and you can strengthen your soft palate to become a more powerful area, not just a flap of fatty skin to vibrate in any passing breath.

This is self-help medicine. It is common sense born out of sound medical reasoning and it should allow you to get rid of snoring and get a decent night's rest.

Chapter Three

How to Cure Snoring

My cure for snoring and the more serious forms of snoring, such as sleep apnoea, is by natural means. It is not alternative medicine. It is sound, normal, medical treatment of the conditions which cause these problems.

I saw a sixty-year-old man who had snored on and off for ten years, but for the last two years his snoring was loud and continuous and his wife was having difficulty getting a full night's sleep. All the usual tensions had built up. She was tired and resentful. He was irritated by her complaints. He felt he slept perfectly well all night.

She said he had become short-tempered and irritable. She said she lay awake worrying that she couldn't get to sleep when he snored. She had got to the stage when she had decided to move into another room to sleep. She told me she realized that this might put a strain on their marriage. They had always had a good sex life together and if she decamped every night, this would stop. That was why she had put up with his snoring for so long. She also confessed that she was afraid to move into another room because when her husband had episodes where he seemed not to be breathing at all, she was afraid he was dying. She felt she might be in time to do something if the episodes became too long. Already, she used to dig him in the side if they were really protracted, she said. That seemed to wake him up with a start and a snort of air. Her love and concern for him were obvious. Her exasperation, born of lack of sleep, was also undeniable. It was clear that though he had come to see me, his wife had insisted he come.

Otherwise healthy, he had gained weight slowly through the years and was, when I saw him, about a stone and a half overweight. His blood pressure was also a little raised, almost certainly due to the extra weight he had put on.

A cassette recording of his nightly snores shattered his belief that he slept soundly and did not need help. We discussed the problems he faced.

As his snoring became worse and he continued to have more and more periods when he did not get breath into his lungs, his brain stem centres might become used to poor oxygen and raised carbon dioxide levels, I told him. His blood cells would increase in number to try to carry more oxygen to his tissues. This would only put an added strain on his heart.

His blood pressure was already slightly raised, I reminded him, and every time he woke or almost woke, choking, his blood pressure would leap to even higher levels with the stress. This could be happening up to 300 times a night. His tape recording convinced him of this. He heard himself struggling for air again and again.

I am not surprised that most heart attacks occur within two hours of wakening. It always seems to me that if a man has had that sort of night, his heart must be exhausted.

It is not surprising, either, that those with asthma or chronic obstructive airways disease who snore seriously and tend towards sleep apnoea are especially at risk of serious respiratory failure.

I did not tell my patient these serious *sequelae*. He was just interested to learn about the causes of snoring and to try to widen his upper throat and strengthen his soft palate by exercise. He was not interested in surgery on an area which was apparently normal.

He went on a diet to lose weight and started the exercises that I have listed in Chapter 5. He sang through them every morning in the car on his way to work.

I talked to him also about the part his diaphragm played in his breathing while he was in rapid eye movement sleep. This also was news to him and he fully realized that being over-weight did not help its action. He started to do exercises to build it up as well, so that when it was the only muscle working to pull air into his lungs it would also be more effective.

Convincing a person that they have a prob-lem caused by lack of muscle usage is half the battle. Both this patient and his wife were convinced. They returned to tell me that the treatment had worked. He was by now down to just about the normal weight for his height and build, but the change had come after he had lost four kilos. His wife described how dramatic the change had been.

One night she had woken to hear him breathing quietly beside her. It was unbeliev-able, she said; the peace; the quiet. She waited for his snoring to restart. It did not. He rolled over and continued to breathe quietly. She turned and fell asleep without a problem. The next night was the same. Occasionally his breathing deepened and she thought, 'Here it comes again.' But it never did.

In exercising his upper throat and soft palate at a time when he was losing weight he had preferentially gained muscle and lost fat deposits in this area, just as distance runners in training gain muscle and lose fat on their limbs and body with exercise and weight control.

For him there was an added bonus. With weight loss, his blood pressure had returned to normal. He needed no medication for it. He had cured the rise himself.

This success story is repeatable for you if this is the cause of your snoring.

What I was particularly pleased about was that he had lost the episodes of sleep apnoea that his wife described so clearly when she said he seemed to stop breathing for a while then wake with a snort.

Interestingly, she returned to tell me that her sleep pattern changed once her husband had stopped snoring. 'I thought I was sleeping less because I was getting older,' she said. 'But now I sleep for longer periods at a time and I don't wake early.'

She had not realized how often she was being wakened by his snoring.

Far from being a condition from which there is no getting better, the brain, given a normal supply of oxygen and normal withdrawal of carbon dioxide, can obviously return to its normal reactivity. The slowing of reaction to the build-up of carbon dioxide that sleep apnoeic people have and which dulls their reaction to a low oxygen supply can be reversed, it seems, especially if the condition is tackled early.

I believe it is even more important not to start to snore. Like not letting your legs get so weak from disuse that you find you cannot enjoy a decent walk in the country; like keeping yourself in trim for life, you should not allow the muscles in your upper throat and soft palate to wither from lack of use.

You will find a spin off if you keep these muscles in good trim. Some of the fibres of the muscles which lift your soft palate have their origin on the eustachean tube, that little tube from your middle ear to your throat. This is the tube that blocks when you go up or down in a plane and can give you earache and a feeling of deafness. My singing exercises so work the muscles in this area that the eustachean tube seems to benefit from them and, if it blocks, a strong soft palate muscle can pull it open easily with a good yawn.

Will these exercises cure all forms of snoring?

No, they will not.

It is therefore essential before you start to do them that you get a simple general check-up from your doctor. He can make sure that your problem does not lie elsewhere.

I should mention other aids that complement my exercises. There is no doubt that lying on your back does increase the possibility of snoring. Your soft palate is then drawn back by its own weight, as is your lower tongue area. Lying on your side is a better position. Then, the natural tone of the muscles in this area works for you as does gravity.

A V-shaped pillow that lies under your head and whose wings keep you on your side is often a great help. If you have already some problems with your heart and your breathing and have to sleep on high pillows, make sure you don't slip down to lie flat on your back.

A bed that bends to keep you in a sitting position may be worth looking at.

Sewing tennis balls into the back of your pyjamas has never seemed to me a very good idea. You are woken every time you turn and it is essential at night to be able to turn to lie on both sides. You can do this more easily with a V pillow.

There are many tips that can help snorers: for instance, if you are a hay fever sufferer, sleep with your window closed to prevent the pollen blowing in in the early morning.

Chapter Four

The Diaphragm

When you are in rapid eye movement sleep your diaphragm is the only muscle causing you to breathe.

By day and in the other parts of sleep, the main muscles that help you breathe are the intercostal muscles that lie between your ribs. They raise the ribs, especially in the lower rib area, and evert their lower border, thus increasing the chest cavity and pulling air into the lungs. They even have some place in contracting the chest cavity to help you breathe out. If you put your hands on your lower ribs and breathe in you will feel this happening.

When you need to breathe more forcibly, you set your shoulders and your upper chest muscles come in to play, helping your intercostal muscles expand your chest to pull air in. Breathing out is mainly performed by relaxation of these muscles, narrowing the chest cavity and squeezing air out of the lungs, although the intercostal muscles and upper chest muscles can help here too. (This is why asthmatics find it easier to breathe in than to breathe out. Most of their muscle power drags air into their contracted lung passages. The resistance the lungs provide if their air passages are in spasm makes it difficult to get the air pushed out again, as simple relaxation of the muscles around the chest is not sufficient to overcome the resistance within the lungs.)

But in rapid eye movement sleep, none of this happens. The intercostal muscles lie paralysed, as do the upper chest muscles. The weight of your chest is supported by the bones of your rib cage, not by the elastic muscles between them.

Your diaphragm is the only muscle that moves except for those round your eyes. Your diaphragm keeps you breathing. It is, at this time, the muscle you rely on for your survival. You really should keep your diaghragm in good working order.

How can you do this? By exercising it regularly. Any muscle improves its action and increases in size and contractility with regular, full usage.

To understand how to exercise let me tell you about your diaphragm. It lies like a horizontal sheet separating your chest contents, your lungs and heart, from your abdominal contents, such as your liver, stomach and bowels. Through it run all the passages from chest to abdomen, such as your gullet, and the blood vessels from your lower body going and coming to your heart. In shape it is a little like a fan, with its handle hanging down to the back. It has attachments to your lower spine, which rise like the handle of the fan to open out into the sheet that separates chest from abdomen. This horizontal fan is attached to the internal circumference of the lower chest wall, from centre front, right round. It lies like a domed tent, convex towards the chest.

Because it is formed from the meeting of two folds of embryonic tissue, one from the front and one from the back, it may on occasion have overlarge gaps for structures like the gullet to pass through. Sometimes it is possible for part of the stomach to slide up into the chest area and then we say that you have a diaphragmatic hernia. The treatment for this, if surgery is not contemplated, is diaphragmatic exercises and to sleep with your bed head raised four inches so that you lie flat but sloping down from head to toes. This way, the weight of your stomach keeps it and your other abdominal contents in your abdomen where they should be.

Many of my patients think they do this by sleeping on raised pillows. This does not work. It folds your body up at the waist, puts pressure on your abdomen and so forces its contents up through any hernia all night. This may lead to disturbed sleep, abdominal discomfort and, if you are a snorer, it does not help your diaphragm work unimpeded. However, this is not such a common condition and usually your diaphragm is complete. Its dome is mostly made from fibrous tissue to which are attached the muscles which arise all round the lower chest circumference.

When these muscles contract, the dome is pulled down towards the abdomen, the chest cavity is increased and the lungs are forced to expand to fill the space. In short, you breathe in. When the diaphragmatic muscles relax, your stomach contents tend to push back into place and your chest cavity gets smaller, your lungs are contracted and you breathe out.

Because of your liver, lying under the right dome of your diaphragm, the descent of the left side tends to be greater at each breath. (This may be why we tend to sleep more upon our right side, not so much to keep the weight of our body off our heart but so that breathing is fuller with less effort, especially in rapid eye movement sleep.)

Like all muscles attached to fibrous central areas, the diaphragm, and indeed the soft palate, which has a similar structure, tends to deteriorate with lack of use, leaving only the non-contractile fibrous area. It is therefore necessary for you to build the muscle that surrounds your diaphragm so that when it is the only piston for your breathing, it is a powerful one.

The diaphragm takes part in all expulsive acts of the body. Before you sneeze, cough, laugh, cry, vomit, pass urine or faeces, you take a big breath and set your diaphragm as a springboard. You can feel the downward movement of your abdominal contents from the V between your ribs as you breathe in if you are using your diaphragm.

Too often you go through the day just breathing shallow breaths in and out that scarcely move your diaphragm at all. This is especially so if you are overweight and your abdomen is already distended with fat.

To exercise the diaphragm, breathe with the diaphragm. The exercises in the next chapter will tell you how. But any action that makes the diaphragm work is good. Playing a wind instrument, or any instrument that you blow, makes you work your diaphragm. Bagpipers have excellent diaphragmatic muscles; so do oboeists. To build up their diaphragms, singers take a huge breath in and let it out in short puffs as if they were laughing, or against their closed lips as if they were playing a trumpet. You will help to build your diaphragmatic muscle when you sing my exercises, especially when you use the sound 'Ho'.

Chapter Five

Exercises

If you are overweight you will get most benefit from these exercises if you also lose weight. You will then lose the fat that surrounds the throat and lies in the soft palate and be left with a wider, muscular throat and well-toned soft palate.

Exercise 1: strengthening the diaphragm

Find a comfortable chair or lie down. Do not exercise standing up as you may feel faint from over-breathing and perhaps run the risk of falling.

1. Lay your hand on the middle of your upper stomach area in the V below your ribs.

2. Breath in, trying to push your hand out. Don't use the front of the stomach muscles.

3. Keep trying a few breaths at a time. Breathe in, hold the breath then breathe out slowly, controlling the breath with the diaphragm.

Do this three times every morning and at night before going to sleep.

Exercise 2: short puffs

1. Breathe in in short puffs, then

2. breathe out again through pursed lips, as if you are playing a trumpet in little puffs.

Last thing at night it is a wonderfully relaxing exercise to take a deep breath in and let it out slowly. Let your worries drift out of your mind as you exhale.

These two exercises should be repeated every day.

Exercise 3: gargling

Keep your upper throat in good condition by

gargling every night to wash away the dust of the day that you have breathed in.

1. Use a very weak solution of ordinary salt and water. It should not taste saltier than soup, just brackish and no more, so that if you swallow it, it does not make you feel sick.

2. If you find it difficult to gargle, after you have done your teeth and washed your mouth out, drink half a cup of lukewarm water. That will also wash the tonsil bed area.

Do this regularly and you may find you are less likely to get chronic throat infections.

Exercise 4: smiling

Singers brighten their expression and almost smile before they start to sing. You should do the same before starting these exercises.

1. Try tightening your cheeks and around your eyes in a little smile. Tighten your upper lip and pull the sides of your mouth up; crinkle up your cheeks and beside your eyes.

2. Let your nostrils flare and your eyebrows rise slightly. You are aiming for a look of surprised delight.

3. Relax.

You should have felt the muscles in the back of your nose and upper throat become taut with this exercise if you did it correctly.

Exercise 5: relaxing the throat

1. Stick your tongue out and down to try to touch your chin.

2. Push, push and feel the back of your throat widen and relax.

3. Rest now and feel the warmth in your throat muscles that this exercise brings.

Exercise 6: to check that your nasal passages are clear

1. Shut the right nostril by placing a finger from your right hand gently against it and breathe in smoothly through your left nostril.

2. Change hands, close off the left nostril and breathe slowly out through the right. Relax.

3. Now breathe in through the right nostril and out through the left.

4. If you feel a blockage you should get it checked by your doctor. If not, you will notice, as you continue my singing exercises, that you will begin to feel more space in the passage behind your nose.

Exercise 7: yawning

Now yawn, a comfortable yawn, not too wide. You are not trying to dislocate your jaw, just allowing your soft palate to try to lift and your upper throat to relax.

At first you will scarcely feel any movement in your soft palate and throat, but as you continue you will be able to lift your soft palate and feel your throat become wider and firmer.

These check exercises are a good monitor of how you are doing. It may be that if you cannot lose weight and do not succeed with the exercises you may have to use a continuous positive airways pressure machine. These exercises can only have helped to make its use more effective.

You are now ready to start my singing exercises.

Singing Exercises

Sing these tunes as loudly as you can.

Don't shout.

Hold the tune but sing strongly to work the muscles in your throat and soft palate.

To begin with sit to sing so that you don't feel faint from the over-breathing of taking in a big breath at the beginning of each line.

Practise each tune at least once a day.

Enjoy the songs.

Self-assessment

Look in a mirror before you start and say 'Ah'. You will get a good idea of how little your soft palate moves. Try this again weekly. After a month you should see a significant difference in your ability to lift your soft palate. Your throat, too, should feel wider and stronger.

To begin with, your upper throat may feel quite tender after a full set of exercises. If this happens, do slightly less the next day but continue to do them regularly, building up each day until you are able to do them all without discomfort.

A month of these exercises and you will feel improvement. They should be continued for life if you get benefit from them.

Singing Exercise 1

For your first exercise, you are going to use the vowel sounds, 'Yah' and 'Ah', sung to the tune of 'Bobby Shaftoe'.

1. Say these sounds now, one after the other.

2. Say them strongly. Feel your soft palate rise with the sound of 'Yah' and 'Ah' as you do when you yawn.

3. Let your mouth open comfortably wide when say 'Yah' and the back of your tongue move down and forward to pull the back of

your upper throat open. Do the same for 'Ah'.

4. Breathe in at the beginning of each line. Try to use your diaphragm and the muscles round your lower chest wall. Don't lift your shoulders to get breath in.
Remember, one song and then a pause or you may feel faint from unaccustomed overbreathing. Many choir singers who stand to sing feel faint even after years of practice, so sing these exercises sitting to begin with and you won't have any trouble.

5. Sing it through three times, first to 'Yah', then to 'Ah', then once more to 'Yah'. Allow yourself to sing louder each time.

6. Then rest.

'Bobby Shaftoe'

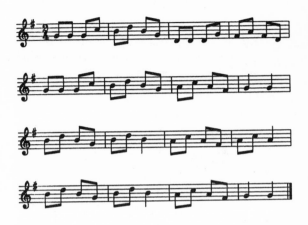

Sing this through using the sound 'YAH' for each note.
Then sing it through using the sound 'AH'.
Sing it through again really loudly using 'YAH'.

Singing Exercise 2

We'll use 'Ho' and 'Hee' for the second exercise. Sing these sounds to the well-known hymn tune 'Guide me, O thou Great Jehovah'. Remember to take a breath before each line.

1. Sing the first verse to 'Ho'. Feel the sound making a huge cave in your upper throat

and your soft palate lifting with each sound.

2. Sing 'Hee' to the second verse. This widens the throat side to side and stretches the soft palate. Don't forget to smile with this verse and feel the muscles behind your nose stretched.

3. Sing it a third time good and loud to 'Ho'.

4. Then relax.

'Guide me, O thou Great Jehovah'

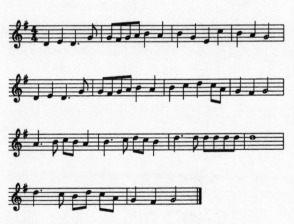

Sing this through using the sound 'HO' for each note.
Then sing it through using the sound 'HEE'.
Sing it through again, loudly, using 'HO'.

Singing Exercise 3: humming

1. Shut your lips, incline your head a little forward and make a big cave in your mouth and throat. Let your tongue lie behind your lower teeth.

2. Now hum as loud as you can. You will feel your upper throat muscles working if you are doing it correctly. We'll use the tune 'My love is like a red, red rose'.

3. Hum it through once, then sing it through to 'Yah', and then hum it again.

4. Don't forget to breathe in before each line and remember to pause before each verse so you don't over-breathe and feel faint.

'My love is like a red, red rose'

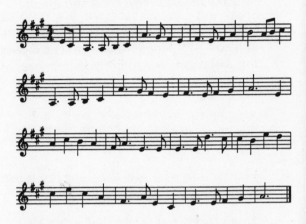

Hum this through making separate humming noises – 'HMN', 'HMN', 'HMN' – for each note. Hum as loudly as you can.
Sing it through again, using the sound 'YAH' to relax your throat.
Then hum it through again, strongly.

Singing Exercise 4

'Good King Wenceslas' is a splendid tune to sing 'Ho' to and you can repeat the exercise of 'Ho' and 'Hee' to it.

1. Sing a verse through to 'Ho' first, then to

'Hee' and then 'Ho' again and remember to make the last verse good and loud.

2. If you feel that your throat and soft palate are tired and strained, do fewer exercises for a day or two until you are free of discomfort.

'Good King Wenceslas'

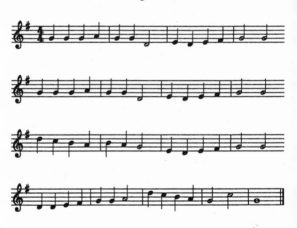

Sing this through using the sound 'HO' for each note.
Then sing it through using the sound 'HEE'.
Sing it through again, loudly, using 'HO'.
Finish off by humming it strongly if you like.

Singing Exercise 5

1. Sing 'Yah' to the tune 'Early One Morning'.

2. Do it staccato, with short sharp sounds.

3. Now sing it again legato to 'Ah', with the notes joined together. The legato sounds are wonderfully relaxing.

4. Then sing it through again to the sound 'Ye'. Make them short, explosive sounds to lift your soft palate and pull your upper throat open.

'Early One Morning'

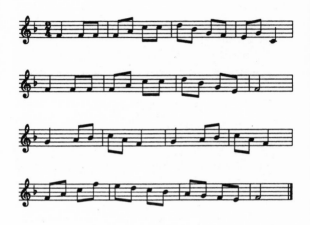

Sing this through using the sound 'YAH' for each note.

Sing it staccato, making the sound short and almost 'YE', 'YE'.
Sing it through again, legato, using 'AH', joining some of the notes together.
Sing it again to 'YE'.

There are other tunes you can sing these sounds through to with benefit. 'Lavender's blue, Dilly Dilly, Lavender's green' goes well to 'Hee' and to humming. I often sing the twenty-third psalm tune 'Crimond' to 'Ho'. I love the tune and the words sing in my mind.

'Love divine, all loves excelling', to the tune that used to be the German national anthem, is great to hum.

You will find other tunes of your own to sing these vowels to. Just remember to use all the sounds and to sing them to tunes with lots of 'jumps' in the music so that your soft palate and upper throat get good exercise.

Never overstrain your voice. You are trying to build muscle where very little muscle exists, so the process must be slow and steady. Think of it as you would athletic training. To begin with, unused muscles give pain on very little activity, but with continuing gentle increase in activity they become strong and active and remain so while you continue to keep them exercised.

I found the added advantage that my singing voice improved immensely. It was a bonus to stopping snoring.

Aim to build up to doing at least twenty minutes' singing a day. You can do it in your bath, in your car driving to work, in your lunch hour wandering in the park.

You can do your routine in short, single tunes or all together in one twenty-minute work-out; but to get the most benefit try to sing for extended periods rather than just one song at a time. Later on, when you find it works, you may even want to sing longer than twenty mintues at a time. That is fine so long as your upper throat does not feel overworked. These are testing exercises if you do them correctly. Professional singers aim to do them for about twenty minutes a day and I recommend that you aim to do the same.

Chapter 6

Case Histories

Case History 1

'I need sleeping pills', said my first patient of the morning. 'Strong ones.'

Nowadays, these are fighting words.

'Why?' I wasn't giving an inch.

'My husband snores and I can't sleep.'

'So what about ear plugs or sleeping in a separate room?' It did not sound too difficult a victory. How wrong I was. She went mad.

'What do you think I have been doing these last ten years and more? What do you think it is like, night after night with a buzz saw in your house? What do you think I feel like every morning as I drag myself to work? What do you think it does to him knowing and seeing what I look like every morning?'

I was routed. She had problems. It was a relief to her to pour it all out. Somewhere, a dam had burst.

She had married her tall, handsome rugby-playing husband twenty years ago. They had met at the local club. Her brother played on the wing, her husband in the boiler house in the second row. She clearly still loved him, but the overlay of exasperation was obvious. When he stopped training the beef went on. His collar size leapt to 18 and he started snoring. At first she could get the noise to stop by nudging him. He snored only when lying on his back. A sharp dig in the ribs made him turn over.

'Sometimes if I just hissed, "Don't Snore", it was enough.'

It wasn't enough for long. First it became the family joke. Then, as night after night of restless sleep affected her, she became less tolerant.

Big and amenable, he tried sewing a tennis ball in the back of his pyjamas.

'That just woke him up as well.'

Then they tried the nose stretchers, the chin straps and separate rooms. Nothing helped. The noise he made echoed through the house.

'He needs a stone castle with a dungeon bedroom.' She was only half in fun. 'An ordinary house is too small to hold him and me.'

His doctor had found the problem amusing. He also snored, he confessed. His wife complained too. Sleeping pills would not help. A constant positive pressure machine might, or he could refer him to an ear, nose and throat specialist who could try a series of laser treatments to his soft palate to try to toughen it up to prevent snoring.

'He came home so miserable and ashamed,' she said. 'He couldn't face sleeping in a mask, all hot and sweaty, or having his soft palate burned. He's a big softy really and my heart bled for him. I couldn't insist. That was when I moved into the back room.'

'What did he think of that?'

'He didn't like it. He felt ashamed. I felt lost. We had been together at night for so long I missed him terribly.'

'No hot water bottle?'

'Worse,' she muttered. 'No sex. Or sex by appointment only.'

This is a common story amongst family partnerships with a snorer. It becomes worse if there are children who are also kept awake, especially when exam time appears and a good night's sleep is essential to a good result.

'If we had children I think I would have insisted he had surgery', she said, following my thought. 'As it's only me who suffers, I put up with poor nights. I snatch a nap whenever I can but I know I am not the live wire at work I used to be. I guess my workmates put it down to my age. But now I get up so exhausted I just feel I need a few nights' real sleep, the sort I used to enjoy.'

'Why now?'

She looked hang dog but clearly had to get it off her chest. 'I have begun to hate him. I used to worry about him. Now I worry about me. I get so resentful when that sound starts and I know I will never get to sleep. I just want to hit him. He knows it too. We never fought. Now we are saying things to each other that are hard and horrid. We don't mean them deep down, at least I don't think we do. But some days I would just give up and leave him and feel thankful for a quiet night.'

I explained the causes of snoring. She knew them already. 'My husband's doctor says his throat has narrowed with him gaining weight and his soft palate is floppy.'

I told her my exercises were designed for people like her husband. He might have to lose weight but if he really sang the exercises every

53

day he should see a difference in a month. I made a bargain. If he had not stopped snoring in three months, I would prescribe a week's sleeping pills, for her. She said it was a deal and went off with the list of songs to sing and the sounds to sing them to. As they were all well known to her, there was no problem.

Not one to bother her doctor unnecessarily she wrote to thank me for 'ending over twenty years of snore-disturbed sleep'.

I know from experience the joy of two people released from the exhaustion that snoring causes. He would sleep deeper and wake fit and active; so would she. More important, her resentment would melt and their relationship would go back to the happy days before he started to snore.

Case History 2

I was going on television in London to talk about using singing exercises to widen the upper throat and strengthen the soft palate to stop snoring. The show was 'Capital Women'; the presenter, Anneke Rice. She was going to produce a married couple where one partner snored. They could discuss the problems with me. When I arrived at the studio, they had not turned up. A telephone call to the producer explained that the chap had snored so badly the night before that his partner had got no sleep. She was cross. He became annoyed at her irritation and they had such a colossal row that they refused to come on the show together.

This is typical of the family misery that snoring causes. At least they had the courage to say that snoring was their problem. Not everyone does. One couple I knew did not.

'I knew he couldn't stop snoring,' she told me, 'so I never complained. The noise wasn't too bad most nights. It was just like going to bed with a large purring tiger. He didn't snore when we were first married. I suppose we both put on weight and became a little less active. He used to tease me about my snoring occasionally. I know I waken with a snort if I lie on my back. I always try to sleep on my side, put the pillows in a V to help me and all that, but sometimes I just seem to slip round. It does annoy me when he talks about it, especially in front of friends, so I don't give it him back. It would just cause trouble and I love him too much to rock the boat for a loss of sleep. Sometimes I give him a nudge and the sound stops for long enough for me to get back to sleep. He never notices.'

She told me that she had seen my method of stopping snoring with singing exercises and had decided to try them.

'My problem is that I can't sing in tune.'

'It doesn't matter,' I told her. 'Just sing good and loud and as tunefully as you can. The songs are well known. You can make a stab at them.'

'I did better than that,' she said. 'I asked my husband to sing along. He can sing in tune and it is more fun singing with him.'

'So where did you do this?'

'In France on holiday, actually. We both wanted to lose a bit of weight so we watched what we ate and took lots of exercise. The place was as flat as a pancake so we hired bicycles and peddled about, singing. What the locals thought I do not know, but singing along on a bicycle brought lots of friendly smiles as we passed.'

'Did it work?'

'Brilliant,' she said. 'After the first two weeks he said I had not snored, but that was probably coincidence because I don't snore regularly, just when I lie on my back. What was amazing was that one night I woke. It was pitch dark and there wasn't a sound from the next bed. I thought he had gone to the bathroom and waited for him to come back. He didn't. I thought, "Oh God, he's dead". I jumped up and pushed him. He complained. I scarcely knew what to say. He had stopped snoring, just like that. One night he was a snarling tiger and the next, silence, and the next and the next. He did not snore again. The funny thing was that, though he had lost a little weight, he had not got down to his ideal when it happened. It was as if the weight had gone off the parts of his throat that he had concentrated on exercising.'

'That happens,' I said. 'Others have said the same to me.'

'Well, it was quite a surprise.'

'Welcome, I hope?'

'More than welcome. My sleep had become fitful. I knew this happened in old age and put it down to that. It's not true. I'm not old yet. Once he stopped snoring I returned to sleeping through the night. He must have been waking me and I didn't know it. No more cat naps for me during the day. It's great. What's more, when we returned from holiday by plane I found that my ears did not block in the way they usually do. It had to be something to do with the exercises. When I yawned they cleared at once: no pain, no fuss.'

'That'll be right enough,' I told her. 'The muscle fibres of the soft palate take off from around the eustachian tube. If you have built up those muscles with my exercises you will have much more control of the eustachian tube and be able to pull it open to relieve the pressure that builds up in the middle ear on landing and taking off.

'If you and your husband keep on singing, even ten minutes or twenty minutes a day, and keep an eye on your weight, you should never return to your snoring habit.'

'It won't be so easy now we are back at work.'

'Sing in the car on the way to and from work, sing on the walk to the bus stop, sing in your bath and when you cook supper. You can always fit it in.'

'I suppose so,' she said. 'It's worth doing.'

Case History 3

A patient brought her seven-year-old boy to see me in surgery. 'He needs your singing exercises,' she said. 'He snores dreadfully.'

'How does he sleep?'

'He sleeps well. We don't. He is entirely out for the count even when he is on his knees with his head bent right back on the pillows. It's weird.'

Children do sleep in the knee-elbow position to try to open their throat passageway as wide as possible. This chap was clearly in trouble. I looked in his throat. His tonsils were huge and septic looking. I did not think they would return to a normal size naturally. His case sheet showed he had had many throat and ear infections. I suspected he had a huge pad of adenoidal tissue behind his nose in his upper throat area.

'Singing won't help here,' I told her. 'I am going to refer him to an ear nose and throat specialist. I think he needs his tonsils and adenoids removed.'

Singing won't cure every cause of snoring. In this case, surgery was the cure.

Case History 4

Mr Johnston sang with a local choral society, so he was most interested to hear about a way to cure snoring with singing. He was strictly amateur, had never had singing lessons, but enjoyed singing. His wife did not enjoy his snoring, so he was motivated to try my cure. He wrote to me to say that though he was perhaps a bit overweight, he did not have a lot to lose and he did not think he needed a strict diet. He had, however, started my exercises and found them fun. He did them formally for twenty minutes a day and occasionally, if the mood took him, he would carol away when he was out of earshot of others. He told me he was amazed how stiff and sore his upper throat and soft palate became.

'Take it easy,' I advised. 'You are building muscle and widening your throat. If you were doing sprint training you would not be surprised by legs that ached a bit as you built up muscle. This is exactly the same. Don't practise so long at any one time, and gradually rebuild to the amount you are doing now.'

He did this and rang to tell me that he was absolutely delighted. His singing voice had improved enormously. He had both greater sound and his range had increased.

'But what about your snoring?' This man seemed to have lost the main purpose somewhere.

'Oh, that has stopped. My wife is delighted.

But of course it did not really worry me. What I find so good is the benefit to my voice.'

I was glad they were both happy. Sometimes you do better than you expect.

Case History 5

'My sleeping problem is a great big lump called John,' said one patient. 'I use Dr Scott's *Sound Asleep for Adults* to help me get to sleep. It is a cassette of classical music timed to run at the brain wave rate of peope going to sleep, and takes me with it. It also drowns the sound John makes and that helps too.

'When I read about Dr Scott's cassette to help people stop snoring I bought it for John. He had been diagnosed as having obstructive sleep apnoea by that time and has to sleep with a mask on attached to a constant positive airways pressure machine, which sits humming away by the bed. It is the best we can do at the moment. He does not want to try surgery. The CPAP machine stops him losing oxygen to his brain when he is deep asleep. I understand this and I know I have to put up with his noise and the machine. It's not much fun for him with a sweaty plastic mask over his face at night and his sinuses are often painful as they seem to infect easily. He is naturally happy to sing and followed the exercises with enthusiasm. He said they made him feel great.

'Anyway, after three months he found he could lower the pressure on his constant positive airways pressure machine and still sleep without airway blockage. How much more improvement we will get I do not know. We are both grateful for what we have. If he loses weight and continues singing, who knows. He may return to being able to sleep without a machine attached. The nice thing about singing is that it makes you feel good. It is not like a punishment, which most cures are. It is fun.'

Case History 6

A professional singer of my acquaintance once complained to me that he snored and snored loudly. There was no way that exercising his upper throat was the answer. It was wide and his soft palate well muscled. His problem was in his nose. He had, I thought, become allergic to something in the atmosphere, possibly at work, possibly at home. The lining of his nose was bright red and swollen. It was this swollen tissue that was vibrating to cause his snores. A simple spray cured this, and his snores. He later tracked the allergy down to dust from a new carpet. The problem was solved in the long term as the vacuum cleaner dealt with the dust.

Case History 7

I learned most of the story from Anne. She was constantly in surgery complaining of pain here and there, depression, trouble with her periods and general gloom. It turned out that most of her symptoms were due to chronic sleep deprivation. James, her partner, snored. She was used to a full eight hours' sleep and had not had that for a couple of years.

James had gained weight before the snoring started. He was a captain of industry and he and Anne went out socially a great deal. Rich food, which he enjoyed, as well as the natural diminution in exercise which his increasing responsibility occasioned, had increased his girth. He had less time for his wife's constant complaints of aches and pains and, though they still functioned as a couple at parties, they scarcely spoke at breakfast.

'If we do speak, we quarrel,' she confessed. 'I have spent all night hating him and the noise he makes and resenting that he is asleep and I am not. So by morning I am fit to be tied. There are nights when I wish he would just die.'

'What about him?'

'He is just cross. You wouldn't think he had been asleep all night. He falls asleep after lunch and he has begun to take a drink before we go out to dinner just to get him to the starting blocks.'

'That won't help.'

'It doesn't. He is dozy after supper and cross by the time we get home. We have monumental rows about little things. We were never like that.'

I explained that, though he seemed to fall asleep as soon as his head hit the pillow, James was missing out on the refreshing stages of sleep. His snoring would keep him almost awake all night.

'At least he does not know he is almost awake. For me, the nights are endless.'

'Sleep in another room.'

'If I did that would be the beginning of a break-up. Things are bad enough already. I keep thinking I should leave him. He is not the even-tempered man I used to know.'

I talked to her about the problems of snoring and explained my natural way to stop it with singing exercises. I suggested he see his doctor and have his blood pressure and weight checked. She seemed interested and encouraged.

A year later when I saw her, they had separated.

'Did he try the exercises?' I asked.

'He thought they were silly,' she said. 'He was embarrassed to sing because he does not sing very well. He did not do them.'

You can't win them all.